My Pregnancy Planner

LOADING

This Planner Belongs To:

Name: _____

Address: _____

E-mail: _____

Website: _____

Phone: _____

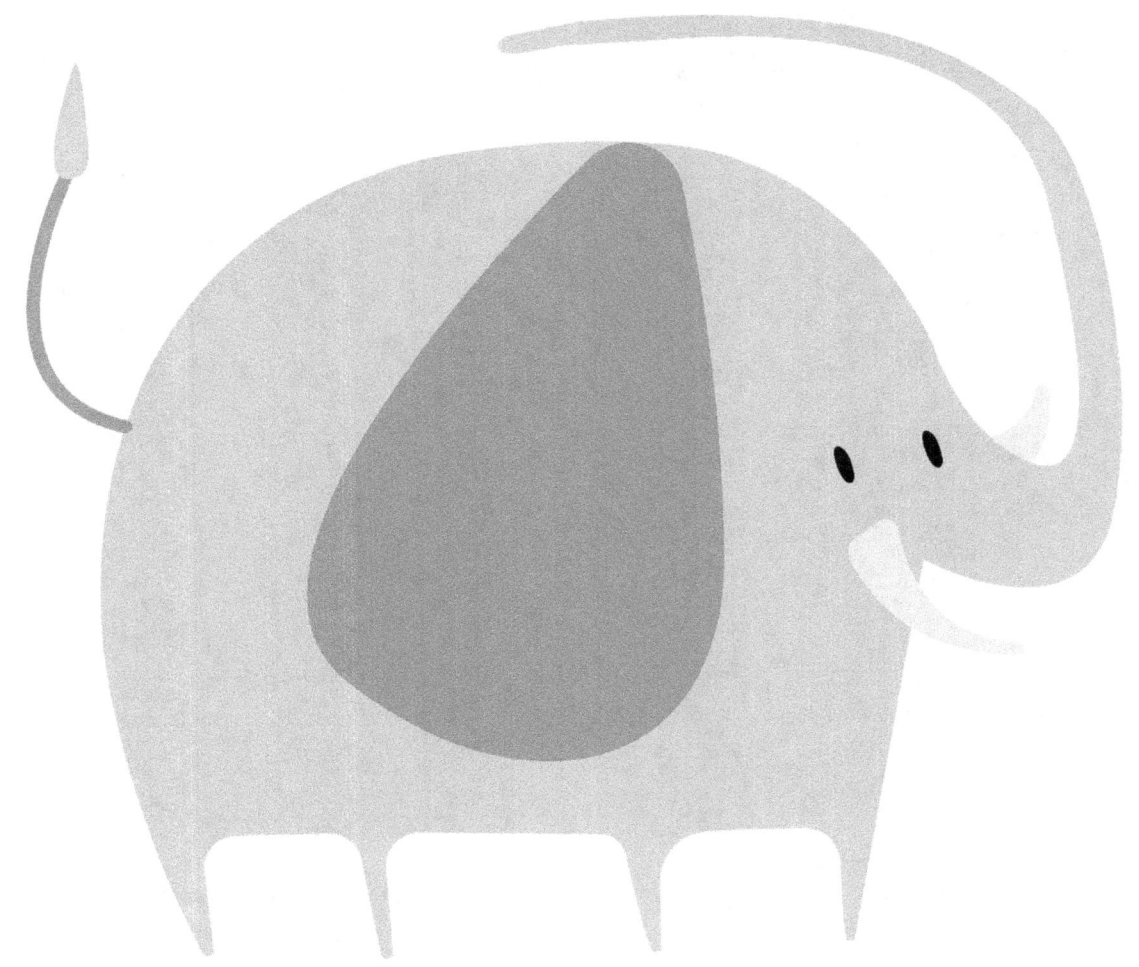

I am .... Years Old

This is my .... Pregnancy

I'm Pregnant

Date I Found Out: ....

How I Revealed Pregancy To My Spouse

....

....

....

....

Spouse's Reaction

....

....

....

Who Did I Tell Next?

....

....

....

....

....

....

Appointment Log

Date:

Doctor Name:

Gestation Age:

Weight:

Blood Pressure:

Fundal Height:

Baby Heart Rate:

Discussion Notes

Appointment Log

Date:

Doctor Name:

Gestation Age:

Weight:

Blood Pressure:

Fundal Height:

Baby Heart Rate:

Discussion Notes

Appointment Log

Date:

Doctor Name:

Gestation Age:

Weight:

Blood Pressure:

Fundal Height:

Baby Heart Rate:

Discussion Notes

Appointment Log

Date:

Doctor Name:

Gestation Age:

Weight:

Blood Pressure:

Fundal Height:

Baby Heart Rate:

Discussion Notes

Appointment Log

Date:

Doctor Name:

Gestation Age:

Weight:

Blood Pressure:

Fundal Height:

Baby Heart Rate:

Discussion Notes

Appointment Log

Date:

Doctor Name:

Gestation Age:

Weight:

Blood Pressure:

Fundal Height:

Baby Heart Rate:

Discussion Notes

Appointment Log

Date:

Doctor Name:

Gestation Age:

Weight:

Blood Pressure:

Fundal Height:

Baby Heart Rate:

Discussion Notes

Appointment Log

Date:

Doctor Name:

Gestation Age:

Weight:

Blood Pressure:

Fundal Height:

Baby Heart Rate:

Discussion Notes

Week: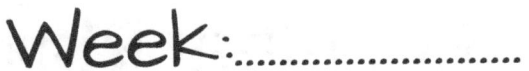

Date:

Baby Is The Size Of:

Current Weight:

Belly Measurement:

Cravings

Aversions

Symptoms

Milestones

What Am I Worried About?

What Am I Excited About?

My Thoughts And Feelings

Meal Planner

Monday

Saturday

Tuesday

Sunday

Wednesday

Geocery List

Thursday

Friday

Journaling

Week:..........................

Date:

Current Weight:

Baby Is The Size Of:

Belly Measurement:

Cravings

Aversions

Symptoms

Milestones

What Am I Worried About?

What Am I Excited About?

My Thoughts And Feelings

Meal Planner

Monday

Tuesday

Wednesday

Thursday

Friday

Saturday

Sunday

Geocery List

Journaling

....

....

....

....

....

....

....

....

....

....

....

....

....

....

....

....

....

....

....

....

Week:..........................

Date:

Current Weight:

Baby Is The Size Of:

Belly Measurement:

Cravings

Aversions

Symptoms

Milestones

What Am I Worried About?

What Am I Excited About?

My Thoughts And Feelings

Meal Planner

Monday

Saturday

Tuesday

Sunday

Wednesday

Geocery List

Thursday

Friday

Journaling

....

....

....

....

....

....

....

....

....

....

....

....

....

....

....

....

....

....

....

....

....

Week: ....

Date: ....

Current Weight: ....

Baby Is The Size Of: ....

Belly Measurement: ....

Cravings

Aversions

Symptoms

Milestones

What Am I Worried About?

What Am I Excited About?

My Thoughts And Feelings

Meal Planner

Monday

Saturday

Tuesday

Sunday

Wednesday

Geocery List

Thursday

Friday

Journaling

Week:.............................

Date:

Current Weight:

Baby Is The Size Of:

Belly Measurement:

Cravings

Aversions

Symptoms

Milestones

What Am I Worried About?

What Am I Excited About?

My Thoughts And Feelings

Meal Planner

Monday

Saturday

Tuesday

Sunday

Wednesday

Geocery List

Thursday

Friday

Journaling

Week:...........................

Date:

Current Weight:

Baby Is The Size Of:

Belly Measurement:

Cravings

Aversions

Symptoms

Milestones

What Am I Worried About?

What Am I Excited About?

My Thoughts And Feelings

Meal Planner

Monday

Saturday

Tuesday

Sunday

Wednesday

Geocery List

Thursday

Friday

Journaling

_____

_____

_____

_____

_____

_____

_____

_____

_____

_____

_____

_____

_____

_____

_____

_____

_____

_____

_____

Week:..........................

Date:

Current Weight:

Baby Is The Size Of:

Belly Measurement:

Cravings

Aversions

Symptoms

Milestones

What Am I Worried About?

What Am I Excited About?

My Thoughts And Feelings

Meal Planner

Monday

Saturday

Tuesday

Sunday

Wednesday

Geocery List

Thursday

Friday

Journaling

Week:..........................

Date:

Current Weight:

Baby Is The Size Of:

Belly Measurement:

Cravings

Aversions

Symptoms

Milestones

What Am I Worried About?

What Am I Excited About?

My Thoughts And Feelings

Meal Planner

Monday

Saturday

Tuesday

Sunday

Wednesday

Geocery List

Thursday

Friday

Journaling

....

....

....

....

....

....

....

....

....

....

....

....

....

....

....

....

....

....

....

....

Week:...........................

Date:

Current Weight:

Baby Is The Size Of:

Belly Measurement:

Cravings

Aversions

Symptoms

Milestones

What Am I Worried About?

What Am I Excited About?

My Thoughts And Feelings

Meal Planner

Monday

Saturday

Tuesday

Sunday

Wednesday

Geocery List

Thursday

Friday

Journaling

_____

_____

_____

_____

_____

_____

_____

_____

_____

_____

_____

_____

_____

_____

_____

_____

_____

_____

_____

Week: ....

Date: _____

Baby Is The Size Of: _____

Current Weight: _____

Belly Measurement: _____

Cravings

Aversions

Symptoms

Milestones

What Am I Worried About?

What Am I Excited About?

My Thoughts And Feelings

Meal Planner

Monday

Saturday

Tuesday

Sunday

Wednesday

Geocery List

Thursday

Friday

Journaling

....

....

....

....

....

....

....

....

....

....

....

....

....

....

....

....

....

....

....

....

....

Week:.........................

Date:

Current Weight:

Baby Is The Size Of:

Belly Measurement:

Cravings

Aversions

Symptoms

Milestones

What Am I Worried About?

What Am I Excited About?

My Thoughts And Feelings

Meal Planner

Monday

Saturday

Tuesday

Sunday

Wednesday

Geocery List

Thursday

Friday

Journaling

_____

_____

_____

_____

_____

_____

_____

_____

_____

_____

_____

_____

_____

_____

_____

_____

_____

_____

_____

_____

Week: ....

Date: _____

Current Weight: _____

Baby Is The Size Of: _____

Belly Measurement: _____

Cravings

Aversions

Symptoms

Milestones

What Am I Worried About?

What Am I Excited About?

My Thoughts And Feelings

Meal Planner

Monday

Saturday

Tuesday

Sunday

Wednesday

Geocery List

Thursday

Friday

Journaling

_____
_____
_____
_____
_____
_____
_____
_____
_____
_____
_____
_____
_____
_____
_____
_____
_____
_____
_____

Week: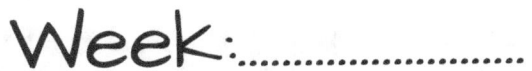

Date:

Current Weight:

Baby Is The Size Of:

Belly Measurement:

Cravings

Aversions

Symptoms

Milestones

What Am I Worried About?

What Am I Excited About?

My Thoughts And Feelings

Meal Planner

Monday

Saturday

Tuesday

Sunday

Wednesday

Geocery List

Thursday

Friday

Journaling

Week:............................

Date: ....

Current Weight: ....

Baby Is The Size Of: ....

Belly Measurement: ....

Cravings

Aversions

Symptoms

Milestones

What Am I Worried About?

What Am I Excited About?

My Thoughts And Feelings

Meal Planner

Monday

Saturday

Tuesday

Sunday

Wednesday

Geocery List

Thursday

Friday

Journaling

_____

_____

_____

_____

_____

_____

_____

_____

_____

_____

_____

_____

_____

_____

_____

_____

_____

_____

_____

_____

Week: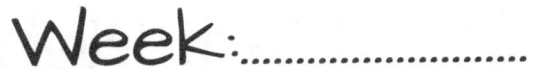

Date:

Baby Is The Size Of:

Current Weight:

Belly Measurement:

Cravings

Aversions

Symptoms

Milestones

What Am I Worried About?

What Am I Excited About?

My Thoughts And Feelings

Meal Planner

Monday

Saturday

Tuesday

Sunday

Wednesday

Geocery List

Thursday

Friday

Journaling

_____

_____

_____

_____

_____

_____

_____

_____

_____

_____

_____

_____

_____

_____

_____

_____

_____

_____

_____

_____

Week: ....

Date: ....

Current Weight: ....

Baby Is The Size Of: ....

Belly Measurement: ....

Cravings

Aversions

Symptoms

Milestones

What Am I Worried About?

What Am I Excited About?

My Thoughts And Feelings

Meal Planner

Monday

Saturday

Tuesday

Sunday

Wednesday

Geocery List

Thursday

Friday

Journaling

Week:.........................

Date:

Current Weight:

Baby Is The Size Of:

Belly Measurement:

Cravings

Aversions

Symptoms

Milestones

What Am I Worried About?

What Am I Excited About?

My Thoughts And Feelings

Meal Planner

Monday

Saturday

Tuesday

Sunday

Wednesday

Geocery List

Thursday

Friday

Journaling

Week:..........................

Date:...

Current Weight:.............................

Baby Is The Size Of:.......................

Belly Measurement:.......................

Cravings

Aversions

Symptoms

Milestones

What Am I Worried About?

What Am I Excited About?

My Thoughts And Feelings

Meal Planner

Monday

Saturday

Tuesday

Sunday

Wednesday

Geocery List

Thursday

Friday

Journaling

_____

_____

_____

_____

_____

_____

_____

_____

_____

_____

_____

_____

_____

_____

_____

_____

_____

_____

Week:............................

Date:

Current Weight:

Baby Is The Size Of:

Belly Measurement:

Cravings

Aversions

Symptoms

Milestones

What Am I Worried About?

What Am I Excited About?

My Thoughts And Feelings

Meal Planner

Monday

Saturday

Tuesday

Sunday

Wednesday

Geocery List

Thursday

Friday

Journaling

_____

_____

_____

_____

_____

_____

_____

_____

_____

_____

_____

_____

_____

_____

_____

_____

_____

_____

_____

_____

Week:........................

Date:

Current Weight:

Baby Is The Size Of:

Belly Measurement:

Cravings

Aversions

Symptoms

Milestones

What Am I Worried About?

What Am I Excited About?

My Thoughts And Feelings

Meal Planner

Monday

Saturday

Tuesday

Sunday

Wednesday

Geocery List

Thursday

Friday

Journaling

_____

_____

_____

_____

_____

_____

_____

_____

_____

_____

_____

_____

_____

_____

_____

_____

_____

_____

_____

Week:................................

Date: ....

Current Weight: ....

Baby Is The Size Of: ....

Belly Measurement: ....

Cravings

Aversions

Symptoms

Milestones

What Am I Worried About?

What Am I Excited About?

My Thoughts And Feelings

Meal Planner

Monday

Saturday

Tuesday

Sunday

Wednesday

Geocery List

Thursday

Friday

Journaling

Week:........................

Date:

Current Weight:

Baby Is The Size Of:

Belly Measurement:

Cravings

Aversions

Symptoms

Milestones

What Am I Worried About?

What Am I Excited About?

My Thoughts And Feelings

Meal Planner

Monday

Saturday

Tuesday

Sunday

Wednesday

Geocery List

Thursday

Friday

Journaling

....

....

....

....

....

....

....

....

....

....

....

....

....

....

....

....

....

....

....

....

....

....

Week:..........................

Date:

Current Weight:

Baby Is The Size Of:

Belly Measurement:

Cravings

Aversions

Symptoms

Milestones

What Am I Worried About?

What Am I Excited About?

My Thoughts And Feelings

Meal Planner

Monday

Saturday

Tuesday

Sunday

Wednesday

Geocery List

Thursday

Friday

Journaling

Week:.........................

Date:

Current Weight:

Baby Is The Size Of:

Belly Measurement:

Cravings

Aversions

Symptoms

Milestones

What Am I Worried About?

What Am I Excited About?

My Thoughts And Feelings

Meal Planner

Monday

Saturday

Tuesday

Sunday

Wednesday

Geocery List

Thursday

Friday

Journaling

Week: ....

Date:

Current Weight:

Baby Is The Size Of:

Belly Measurement:

Cravings

Aversions

Symptoms

Milestones

What Am I Worried About?

What Am I Excited About?

My Thoughts And Feelings

Meal Planner

Monday

Saturday

Tuesday

Sunday

Wednesday

Geocery List

Thursday

Friday

Journaling

_____

_____

_____

_____

_____

_____

_____

_____

_____

_____

_____

_____

_____

_____

_____

_____

_____

_____

_____

_____

Week:...........................

Date:

Current Weight:

Baby Is The Size Of:

Belly Measurement:

Cravings

Aversions

Symptoms

Milestones

What Am I Worried About?

What Am I Excited About?

My Thoughts And Feelings

Meal Planner

Monday

Saturday

Tuesday

Sunday

Wednesday

Geocery List

Thursday

Friday

Journaling

Week: ....

Date: ....

Current Weight: ....

Baby Is The Size Of: ....

Belly Measurement: ....

Cravings

Aversions

Symptoms

Milestones

What Am I Worried About?

What Am I Excited About?

My Thoughts And Feelings

Meal Planner

Monday

Saturday

Tuesday

Sunday

Wednesday

Geocery List

Thursday

Friday

Journaling

_____

_____

_____

_____

_____

_____

_____

_____

_____

_____

_____

_____

_____

_____

_____

_____

_____

_____

_____

_____

Week:........................

Date:

Current Weight:

Baby Is The Size Of:

Belly Measurement:

Cravings

Aversions

Symptoms

Milestones

What Am I Worried About?

What Am I Excited About?

My Thoughts And Feelings

Meal Planner

Monday

Saturday

Tuesday

Sunday

Wednesday

Geocery List

Thursday

Friday

Journaling

Week:...........................

Date: _____

Current Weight: _____

Baby Is The Size Of: _____

Belly Measurement: _____

Cravings

Aversions

Symptoms

Milestones

What Am I Worried About?

What Am I Excited About?

My Thoughts And Feelings

Meal Planner

Monday

Saturday

Tuesday

Sunday

Wednesday

Geocery List

Thursday

Friday

Journaling

_____

_____

_____

_____

_____

_____

_____

_____

_____

_____

_____

_____

_____

_____

_____

_____

_____

_____

_____

Week:..........................

Date: ....

Current Weight: ....

Baby Is The Size Of: ....

Belly Measurement: ....

Cravings

Aversions

Symptoms

Milestones

What Am I Worried About?

What Am I Excited About?

My Thoughts And Feelings

Meal Planner

Monday

Saturday

Tuesday

Sunday

Wednesday

Geocery List

Thursday

Friday

Journaling

Week:..............................

Date:

Current Weight:

Baby Is The Size Of:

Belly Measurement:

Cravings

Aversions

Symptoms

Milestones

What Am I Worried About?

What Am I Excited About?

My Thoughts And Feelings

Meal Planner

Monday

Saturday

Tuesday

Sunday

Wednesday

Geocery List

Thursday

Friday

Journaling

Week:................................

Date:

Baby Is The Size Of:

Current Weight:

Belly Measurement:

Cravings

Aversions

Symptoms

Milestones

What Am I Worried About?

What Am I Excited About?

My Thoughts And Feelings

Meal Planner

Monday

Saturday

Tuesday

Sunday

Wednesday

Geocery List

Thursday

Friday

Journaling

....

....

....

....

....

....

....

....

....

....

....

....

....

....

....

....

....

....

....

....

....

Week: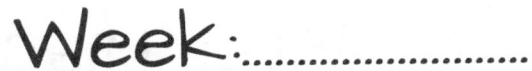............................

Date:

Current Weight:

Baby Is The Size Of:

Belly Measurement:

Cravings

Aversions

Symptoms

Milestones

What Am I Worried About?

What Am I Excited About?

My Thoughts And Feelings

Meal Planner

Monday

Saturday

Tuesday

Sunday

Wednesday

Geocery List

Thursday

Friday

Journaling

Week:....................

Date: ....

Current Weight: ....

Baby Is The Size Of: ....

Belly Measurement: ....

Cravings

Aversions

Symptoms

Milestones

What Am I Worried About?

What Am I Excited About?

My Thoughts And Feelings

Meal Planner

Monday

Saturday

Tuesday

Sunday

Wednesday

Geocery List

Thursday

Friday

Journaling

_____

_____

_____

_____

_____

_____

_____

_____

_____

_____

_____

_____

_____

_____

_____

_____

_____

_____

_____

_____

_____

Week: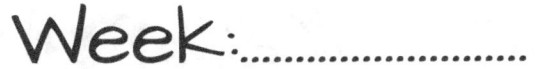

Date: ....

Current Weight: ....

Baby Is The Size Of: ....

Belly Measurement: ....

Cravings

Aversions

Symptoms

Milestones

What Am I Worried About?

What Am I Excited About?

My Thoughts And Feelings

Meal Planner

Monday

Tuesday

Wednesday

Thursday

Friday

Saturday

Sunday

Geocery List

Journaling

_____

_____

_____

_____

_____

_____

_____

_____

_____

_____

_____

_____

_____

_____

_____

_____

_____

_____

_____

Week:...........................

Date:

Current Weight:

Baby Is The Size Of:

Belly Measurement:

Cravings

Aversions

Symptoms

Milestones

What Am I Worried About?

What Am I Excited About?

My Thoughts And Feelings

Meal Planner

Monday

Saturday

Tuesday

Sunday

Wednesday

Geocery List

Thursday

Friday

Journaling

Baby's 1st Ultrasound

Place A Photo of Baby's
First Ultrasound Here!

Date:....................................

Baby's 2nd Ultrasound

Place A Photo of Baby's
Ultrasound Here!

Date:.....................................

Baby's 3rd Ultrasound

Place A Photo of Baby's
Ultrasound Here!

Date:....................................

Week:..............

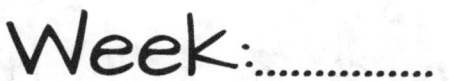

Place A Photo of Yourself,
Or Belly Pics
During Your Pregnancy Here!

Date:....................................

Week:..............

Place A Photo of Yourself,
Or Belly Pics
During Your Pregnancy Here!

Date:.....................................

Week: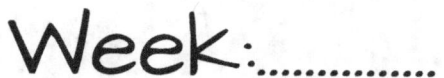...............

Place A Photo of Yourself,
Or Belly Pics
During Your Pregnancy Here!

Date:.................................

Week:...............

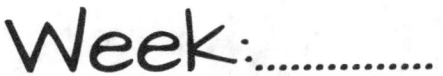

Place A Photo of Yourself,
Or Belly Pics
During Your Pregnancy Here!

Date:...................................

Week:..............

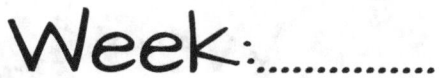

Place A Photo of Yourself,
Or Belly Pics
During Your Pregnancy Here!

Date:...................................

Week:...............

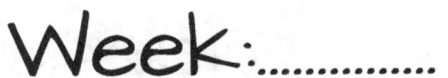

Place A Photo of Yourself,
Or Belly Pics
During Your Pregnancy Here!

Date:....................................

Week:...............

Place A Photo of Yourself,
Or Belly Pics
During Your Pregnancy Here!

Date:..................................

Week:.............

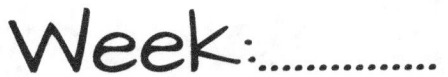

Place A Photo of Yourself,
Or Belly Pics
During Your Pregnancy Here!

Date:....................................

Week:..............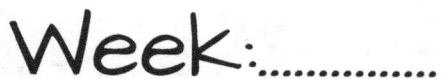

Place A Photo of Yourself,
Or Belly Pics
During Your Pregnancy Here!

Date:....................................

My Birthday Plan

Due Date:

Name: Partner's Name:

Doctor: Hospital:

Planned Delivery Method:

Backup Delivery Method:

Special Notes:

I Want These People To Be Present During Labor/or Birth:

Partner:

Friends:

Relatives:

Doula:

Children:

Notes

Hospital Bag Suggestion List

If you are wondering what to pack in your hospital bag for labor, here are the essentials you should gather together so there's no last-minute rush to fill a suitcase between contractions.

Hospital bag essentials:

- Drivers' license or other identification card
- Insurance card and any hospital paperwork you've filled out
- Your birth plan, if you have one (bring multiple copies to give to your practitioner and various nurses)
- Your phone and a charger
- An outfit for your baby to wear home
- Clothing for you to wear home (think baggy, soft and comfortable!)
- Small tote for extra hospital supplies and any gifts you might receive
- Infant car seat (It should be sized for a typical newborn's weight - and also installed correctly. A few weeks before you're due, install yours and get it inspected by a certified technician, which you can find through the National Highway Traffic Safety Administration.)

Hospital bag checklist for mom:

Personal items

- Hair ties, clips or a headband to keep your hair out of your face as you labor
- Toothbrush, toothpaste and mouthwash
- Hairbrush, comb
- Glasses, contacts and saline solution if you wear lenses
- Lotion, lip balm, deodorant
- Extra-absorbent maxi pads (the hospital will provide them, but you might want to use the brand you're most comfortable with)
- Shampoo, conditioner, face wash, soap, shower gel, makeup and whatever else it takes to make you feel refreshed after delivery
- Massage oils or lotion for labor if you have any you want with you

Clothing

- Extra pairs of underwear suitable for wearing with maxi pads
- Nursing bra and breast pads for any leakage, in case you plan to nurse
- Nightgown or pajamas
- Lightweight bathrobe to throw on if visitors arrive
- Cozy socks with grip soles or slippers
- Cardigan, zip-front fleece or sweatpants in case you get cold

Hospital Bag Suggestion List

Entertainment/food

- Snacks to eat during labor (your own snacks will be limited and must be approved by your practitioner; your partner should pack sandwiches and nutritious nibbles so they don't have to leave your side to find something to eat)
- Snacks for after delivery - don't count on the hospital or birthing center to provide them in the middle of the night (think crackers, granola, carrot sticks, apples)
- Music or headphones that plug into your phone
- Diversions for a long labor, such as a juicy novel, crossword puzzles, magazines, a deck of cards, laptop or handheld electronic games
- A baby care book, like What to Expect the First Year (if you have room to pack it and think you'll have a chance to look at it)
- A baby keepsake book so you can pen some first thoughts and memories

Miscellaneous items

- Your favorite pillow or lightweight blanket to snuggle with
- Your cord blood banking kit, if you're banking your baby's cord blood (if you decide to bank your baby's cord blood at the last minute, you can have the company overnight you a kit or ask the hospital if there are kits available for you to use)
- Any mementos you'll want with you, such as family photos
- Your "who to call" list so you can share or text the good news
- A small basket of goodies for the staff to give along with the birth plan, if you'd like

Hospital bag checklist for baby

Your baby won't need much more than something to wear home and his car seat, but here are a few other items to consider, depending on the weather and the size of your bag:

- Baby lotion, diaper cream and a diaper or two (though the hospital will provide plenty)
- Going-home outfit, including socks or booties
- A receiving blanket and a couple of burp cloths
- Extra layers like a sweater or bunting, plus a knit cap if it's cold out
- A hat with a little brim in case it's sunny

Hospital bag checklist for partners

Labor can be long - and there will be times when your partner doesn't have much to do. Here's what might come in handy:

Personal items:

- Phone and a charger
- Gum, mints, lip balm
- Toothbrush, toothpaste, deodorant, spare contact lenses, glasses and other toiletries
- A travel pillow or bed pillow in case of a cat nap or overnight stay

Hospital Bag Suggestion List

Clothing

- Sweatshirt or jacket for quick runs to the drugstore or deli
- A change of underwear and fresh shirt in case labor goes on - and on
- Pajamas in case of an overnight stay

Entertainment/food

- Snacks - and more snacks, especially ones that keep well (pretzels, trail mix, granola bars)
- Small bills or change for vending machines and the hospital cafeteria
- Reusable water bottle or another beverage (juice, Gatorade)
- A camera and/or video camera, if you have one and want to capture early memories
- Diversions, like a paperback, newspaper, magazines or Sudoku

Hospital Bag Checklist

Baby Name Ideas

Our Top Picks

Dear Baby

Nursery To-Do List

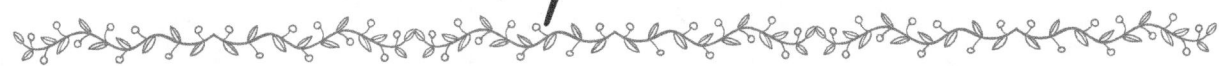

<u>A crib or bassinet.</u> Your baby needs a safe, flat firm sleeping space. Do not put any blankets, pillows, stuffed animals, crib bumpers, decorations or anything else besides a fitted sheet in the crib with your baby. However, under the crib is another story, and that is a great spot for storage.

<u>A crib mattress.</u> Remember, you'll also need to buy a crib mattress to go with the crib! Don't register for just the crib and then forget you'll need the mattress, too. Waterproof mattress protectors (two so that you can change them out) are also good to have.

<u>Crib sheets.</u> You'll need at least three crib sheets since sometimes you need to change the sheets more than once a night due to spit-up and diaper leaks.

A changing table and diaper items. This is a great opportunity to double up and put a changing pad on top of a dresser or other storage. You'll need a caddy (or the top drawer of a dresser) for diapers, wipes and diaper cream, but you don't need a wipes warmer. You do need at least two changing pad covers.

<u>A rocking chair or glider.</u> For feedings (either breastfeeding or bottle feeding) and for rocking to sleep, you do need a spot where you can sit to do this, especially in the middle of the night. The matching footstool isn't essential, though. A nursing pillow (helpful for formula feeding, too) is very good to have, too.

<u>A hamper.</u> When you're changing your baby's outfit on the changing table, you'll want to be able to drop the dirty clothes right into a hamper. You'll want one that doesn't take up too much floor space (think tall and narrow instead of wide and short) and that is easily transported to the washing machine (or with a removable bag for that).

<u>A diaper pail.</u> Next to the changing station, you'll need somewhere to dispose of the dirty diapers. Ideally, something covered and sealed, like a Diaper Genie.

A baby monitor. Unless you are sleeping right next door or in the room and feel confident you'll be awakened by your baby's cries, get a baby monitor so you can be alerted when it's time to go into the nursery for whatever your baby needs. A video monitor isn't essential, but it is definitely very helpful.

<u>Clothing storage.</u> You'll need either a dresser or a closet (or both!) for your baby's clothes.

Nursery To-Do List

What's nice to have in a nursery.

A humidifier. You may not need this, and plenty of babies do fine without one.

Babyproofing items. Of course, these are essential months down the line, but for now, you don't need to worry about any latches or doorknob covers. But if you are struggling to think of things to add to your registry, why not get a jump start on these items now?

Extra diapers. Register for some size 1, 2 and 3 diapers to get a head start. They'll definitely get used, and you never know how big your baby will be when they're born.

Blackout curtains. Any window dressings will do, but blackout curtains will help to make sure your baby isn't woken up by the sun during nap times.

A mobile. Your baby will do just fine without one, though they are really nice to help put them to sleep.

Nursery To-Do List

To-Do List	To Buy List

Baby Shopping List

Ideas And Notes

Ideas And Notes

Ideas And Notes

Ideas And Notes

Ideas And Notes

Ideas And Notes

Thank You!

Pregnancy Journal

so much for trying our Pregnancy Journal!
We'd love to hear from you!

If you've found this to be a good notebook please,

support us and leave a review.

If you have any suggestions or issues with this journal, or if

you want to test some of our latest notebooks

please email us.

Send email to:

pickme.readme@gmail.com

Copyrights
@ 2022
All rights reserved